Anti-Inflammatory Diet

The Ultimate Beginner's Guide Plan & 20+

Proven Recipes To Naturally Heal Your

Inflammation, Treat Immune System, Alleviate

Pain and Restore Your Physical Health

By *Jennifer Louissa*

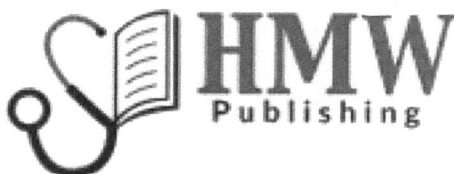

I0222586

HMW
Publishing

For more great books visit:

HMWPublishing.com

Get another book for Free

I want to thank you for purchasing this book and offer you another book (just as long and valuable as this book), "Health & Fitness Mistakes You Don't Know You're Making", completely free.

Visit the link below to signup and receive it:

www.hmwpublishing.com/gift

In this book, I will break down the most common health & fitness mistakes, you are probably committing right now, and I will reveal how you can easily get in the best shape of your life!

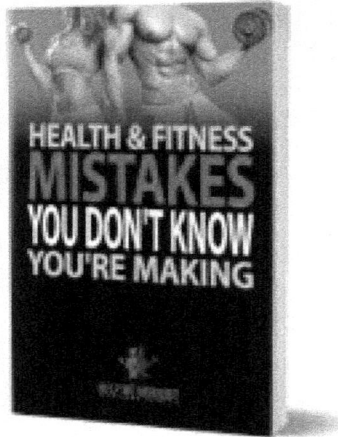

In addition to this valuable gift, you will also have an opportunity to get our new books for free, enter giveaways, and receive other valuable emails from me. Again, visit the link to sign up:

www.hmwpublishing.com/gift

Table of Contents

INTRODUCTION

Every time we think of inflammation, we generally visualize swollen parts of the body such as joints, arthritic limbs, stiff muscles, etc. We have come to associate these with inflammation and something that affects old people. However, inflammation is more than just joint pains, gout, or arthritis. In fact, inflammation can and does affect our entire body regardless of age. It can affect us from the day we are born and until the day we die.

Also, before you get started, I recommend you **joining our email newsletter** to receive updates on any upcoming new book releases or promotions. You can sign-up for free, and as a bonus, you will receive a free gift. Our *"Health & Fitness Mistakes You Don't Know You're Making"* book! This book has been written to demystify, expose the top do's and don'ts and to finally equip you with the information you need to get in the best shape of your life. Due to the overwhelming amount of mis-information and lies told by magazines and self-proclaimed "gurus", it's becoming harder and harder to get reliable information to get in shape. As opposed to having to go through dozens of biased, unreliable and untrustworthy sources to get your health & fitness information. Everything you need to help you has been broken down in this book for you to easily follow and to immediately get results to achieve your desired fitness goals in the shortest amount of time.

Once again, to join our free email newsletter and to receive a free copy of this valuable book, please visit the link and signup now: **www.hmwpublishing.com/gift**

CHAPTER 1 - INFLAMMATION AWARENESS: THE SPOTLIGHT EXAMINATION

Every time we think of inflammation, we generally visualize swollen parts of the body such as joints, arthritic limbs, stiff muscles, etc. We have come to associate these with inflammation and something that affects old people. However, inflammation is more than just joint pains, gout, or arthritis. In fact, inflammation can and does change our entire body regardless of age. It can affect us from the day we are born and until the day we die.

What does Inflammation do to the Body?

Inflammation is the process which the body uses to protect itself as it creates an area of healing within the body. Inflammation usually is characterized by swelling, pain, redness, and a feeling of something hot, but not all inflammation cause symptoms that we can sense or experience.

In contrast to our shared belief that inflammation can only affect those in old age, the sad truth is inflammation can strike anyone regardless of age. Even children can experience swelling in forms of allergies and asthma as well as when they get body injuries. Young adults, too, can suffer from inflammation of various areas of the body including that of the cardiovascular system.

According to a study published in "Jornal de Pediatria," regarding the effect of Fish Oil on cardiovascular risk factors during teenage growth, they discovered that fish oil improves cardiovascular health in slightly overweight teenagers.

Adults similarly suffer from various forms of inflammation and can be prone to even worse swelling as the body ages. Furthermore, there is an increasing incidence of inflammation every year, causing higher deaths attributed to the whole body's inflammation system and this fact is getting out of control.

Whether we are conscious of it or not, we are all experiencing a form of inflammation on a daily basis. However, only a few manage to fully understand the purpose of inflammation and what it serves in our physical body as a form of armed protection. Which is mainly a response triggered by damaged living tissue inside your body and often are not aware of the damage and havoc it created for us when we left it unchecked.

Many can see the redness or the swelling we get upon injury, but we are not aware that it represents only one kind of inflammation, the acute inflammation. Inflammation by itself is a natural process, and healing could not take place in the body without it. Severe inflammation is the body's reaction to injury and helps us in repairing and protecting damaged tissues. It likewise protects us from diseases and illness. This type of inflammation acts as a form of a medic pack to heal the immune system by bringing more nourishment activity to the area where they are needed most.

Inflammation can become dangerous and even deadly once it manifests as chronic inflammation. As the name suggests, this type of inflation is recurring. This medium usually happens when the initial stimulus that leads to acute inflammation continues which means that the body interprets it as unresolved.

This form of inflammation, in nature, is quite sinister as it silently attacks, damaging your tissues without the usual redness, heat, swelling or pain that is usually typically observed in acute inflammation.

Damaged tissue is a classic hallmark of chronic inflammation and often forms fibrous or scar tissue from the tissue which once appeared on the site of repair. Angiogenesis or new blood vessel formation is another hallmark of chronic inflammation, and it plays a significant role in the creation of substantial diseases like cancer.

Chronic inflammation is often associated with autoimmune disorders, from viral and bacterial reactions, allergic reactions, to a host of other diseases and processes such as:

- Allergies

- Multiple Sclerosis

- Crohn's Disease

- Heart Disease

- Alzheimer's Disease

- Cancer

- Cancer

- Obesity

- Atherosclerosis

- Asthma

- Rheumatoid Arthritis

- Diabetes

- Celiac Disease

- As well as many other conditions including other inflammatory conditions like gastritis, tendonitis, endocarditis, and much more.

What Causes the Rise in Inflammation?

As we have mentioned, inflammation is a healthy and natural human process which helps in healing and protecting our body, but the body relies on two essential fatty acids to keep this process in balance within us.

Our body needs nutrients and minerals to stay healthy. Two of the essential elements required by the body to help it produce the chemicals needed which aids in keeping us healthy are Omega 3-6-9 fatty acids. The Omega 3 by itself is seen more often in the organic or supplement section of many stores which is primarily the fatty acid needed, more than omega 6 and 9. This fatty acid can be acquired not only by supplement form but also in healthy fatty foods like eggs of salmon fish, etc.

In proportion, the body utilizes Omega 3 to produce anti-inflammatory chemicals and uses Omega 6 to produce inflammatory compounds. When everything is in the balance, the body can automatically combat pollutants and invaders from outside.

The problem today is the fact that our body is no longer getting a fair proportion of these required nutrients. Our modern lifestyle has drastically increased the amount of Omega 6 that we are consuming while reducing the intake of omega 3 fatty acids. Resulting in an imbalance in our body system because the body needs more Omega 3 than 6 and having Omega 6 by itself acts as a form of toxic to the body.

With the added amount of Omega 6 fatty acids, it causes our body to produce more inflammatory chemicals while the lack of Omega 3 causes it to reduce the production of anti-inflammatory elements.

The result of this imbalance is not only hazardous but fatal in various cases since inflammation builds up in our system daily. Inflammation can likewise attack any tissues within our body which means that it can be accumulated in the cardiovascular system, the respiratory system, skeletal system, or anywhere within our body.

What Triggers It?

Although acute inflammation is usually beneficial, it often results to unpleasant sensations such as the pain of a sore throat or the itching caused by insect bites. Typically, such discomfort appears to be temporary and quickly disappears when the inflammatory response has done its function.

However, there are instances when inflammation can cause harm. When the regulatory mechanism of the inflammatory responses is defective, or its ability to clear damaged tissue and foreign substances is impaired, tissue destruction can occur.

In other cases, a damaged or inappropriate immune response can give rise to a prolonged and damaging inflammatory response. An example of this is hypersensitivity or allergic reaction. Environmental agents like pollen, which usually poses no threat to a person can trigger inflammation and autoimmune reactions. Hence, chronic inflammation is stimulated by the body's immune response against its tissues.

Causes of Inflammation

Factors that trigger inflammation include the following:

- Physical agents

- Chemicals

- Microorganism

- Inappropriate immunological responses

- Tissue death

- Viruses and bacteria

Viruses give rise to inflammation by entering the body and destroying its cells. Bacteria release substances called *"endotoxins"* which can initiate inflammation. Conditions like physical trauma, radiation, frostbites, and burns can damage tissues and likewise bring swelling. Added to these are corrosive chemicals such as acids, alkalis, and oxidizing agents. Inflammation also results when tissues die due to lack of oxygen or nutrients, a condition that is caused by loss of blood flow in the area affected.

Symptoms and Awareness

The four significant primary signs of inflammation are:

- Redness (Latin rubor) – caused when there is dilation of small blood vessels in the area of injury.

- Heat (latin word: calor) – Heat occurs when there is increased blood flow through the area and is being experienced only in areas of peripheral body parts such as the skin. Fever is brought about by medical mediators of inflammation which then contributes to the rise in temperature at the injury.

- Pain (latin word: dolor) – The pain brought by the inflammation is caused in part by the distortion of tissues caused by edema and is also induced by specific chemical mediators of inflammation including bradykinin, prostaglandins, and serotonin.

- Swelling (tumor) also called "edema" and is primarily caused when there is accumulated fluid outside the blood vessels.

Another consequence of inflammation is the loss of functions of the inflamed area, an activity noted by Rudolf Virchow, a German pathologist in the 19th century. The damage can be caused by pain that inhibits mobility either from or as a result of a severe swelling that prevents movement in the area.

CHAPTER 2 – THE ROLE OF FOOD INFLAMMATORY - CAUSING FOODS NO ONE TALKS ABOUT

What one eats matters and the number one way to reduce inflammation risk is through diet. Sugar, dairy, and grains are considered the most significant offenders. However, this does not mean that you have to go completely free of gluten unless you have a Celiac disease. Some people are okay with gluten as long as they cut out wheat but keep rye, barley or spelt-Wheat. The same thing goes for dairy and sugar. The problem occurred when you began to rely on these foods, and you're overeating of them.

When there's inflammation in your body, possible consequences could be heart disease, cancer, acne, and Alzheimer's.

"Our body depends on temporary inflammation to help fight off sudden injuries or infection. However, when the swelling becomes persistent and recurring, the immune system attacks healthy cells, and the process of healing becomes destructive.

Limiting the intake of particular food is not enough. It is essential to eat foods that support the liver as it is in charge of clearing toxins out – greens leafy vegetables, grains, lean proteins, herbs, healthy fats, and from time to time sip healthy organic juice or tea that is low in sugar content. These are nature's contribution to fighting against anti-inflammation crusade.

The Real Culprits

Amy Wechsler, MD., a New York dermatologist believes that the most prominent culprit when it comes to inflammation is stress and not diet!

"Stress signals to the adrenaline glands to release adrenaline which then commandeers blood from the skin and leaving behind a wan, washed-out look."

Stress likewise released other hormones including cortisol which contributes to inflammatory skin disorders such as acne and tensed people are more prone to picking their pimples which exacerbate the inflammatory response.

To prevent inflammation from hurting you, do what you can to avoid stress. You can spend time socializing with friends, sleep and cuddle with your partner, have regular exercises, and even have sex. All these will help you feel less stressed and show visible lasting signs on your skin and psyche.

Though most of the time, "sugar" is pinpointed to be the culprit along with other offenders like dairy, transfat-filled fast foods, and booze, you must be aware that inflammation can make a sneak through any of these seemingly innocent foods that no one seems to mention.

When *Nicholas Perricone, Md.* A pioneering nutritionist and dermatologist wrote his book on anti-inflammation eating; he believed that our body depends contemporary inflammation to help fight off sudden injuries or infection. However, like what had been discussed in the previous chapter, the healer turns into a destroyer when the inflammation becomes chronic and attacks healthy cells by mistake.

Like many health issues, the sugar is considered to be playing a significant role and is singled out as the major offenders though there are others as well. Here are some of the seeming innocent foods that are surprising sources of inflammation that you might need to consider with caution.

Agave

Though the agave plant has been introduced as a worry-free sweetener, it is still full of sugar – with a fructose content of up to 90 percent. According to Dr. Perricone, a known dermatologist, "Sugar suppresses the activity of our white blood cells making us more susceptible to infectious diseases such as flu and colds and even cancer. Sugar overload also causes collagen fibers to lose their strength making skin more vulnerable to sun damage, sagging, and wrinkles.

Frozen yogurt

Frozen yogurts contain sugar and dairy which are considered potential inflammatory culprits. Milk can boost insulin levels and male hormones aside from being a universal allergen which means that it can trigger inflammatory reactions. Nonetheless, not all yogurts are created equal according to Andrew Weil, M.D., director of the Arizona Center for Integrative Medicine at the College of Medicine and an anti-inflammatory evangelist.

Dr. Weil said that some yogurts contain casein (milk protein) which may increase inflammation while others contain specific probiotics that may reduce it. There are also yogurts that contain no dairy at all and use coconut milk instead.

Barley and Rye

These grains are healthy and delicious and don't carry the same effect that refined carbohydrates do regarding sugar spike, but they can likewise spark inflammation in some people. It is due to gluten that especially when you are sensitive to it or if you suffer from Celiac disease. Consumption of barley and rye, either in food or alcohol can cause your issues to flare up. If you got trouble with your joints and aching, these are indications of inflammation.

Seitan:

This vegetable is known as "wheat meat" because it is composed of wheat gluten. We all know that gluten can trigger the immune system. Which causes inflammation of the intestinal that can act and is manifested in bloating, IBS or constipation in some people.

Peanuts

Peanuts, like milk, are common allergens and often people are sensitive or allergic which set off an inflammatory response in the body while it struggles to combat the presence of a foreign body. Peanuts are also prone to molds and fungus which can likewise result in inflammatory reactions, according to Wood. So instead of peanuts, choose raw organic almond or other tree nuts and butter.

Seasoning Mixes

We all love seasoning mixes as they add natural to flavor and provide an excellent short-cut to our cooking activities, but they usually contain artificial coloring which can disrupt hormonal function leading to inflammation and elevated sugar content. To acquire the same taste without all the bad stuff, you use instead a combination of cayenne pepper cracked pepper, apple cider vinegar with sea salt.

CHAPTER 3 – EATING YOUR WAY OUT OF PAIN AND INFLAMMATION: GOOD RULES FOR AN ANTI -INFLAMMATORY DIET

Unlike any other diets, the Anti-Inflammatory diet is not for losing weight – though people can lose weight on it – nor should it stay for a limited period. Instead, it is a way of choosing what you should eat based on a scientific knowledge of how these foods can help you maintain optimum health.

Along with protection from inflammation, this natural diet will provide you with a physical energy and adequate supply of vitamins, minerals, protective phytonutrients, and the essential fatty acids dietary fiber. You can adapt your meal recipes to these anti-inflammatory diet principles.

General Guide Rule

- Eat a variety of fruits and minerals.

- Aim for as many fresh foods as possible.

- Minimize intake of fast and processed food.

Intake of Calories

- These previously mentioned foods are examples of not so good carbs for inflammation, but that doesn't mean there are no good carbs. A good carbohydrate example can be from beans, fish, eggs, vegetables growing above ground and natural fats (like butter). Avoid sugar and starchy foods (like bread, pasta, rice, beans, and potatoes).

- If you consume healthy carbs, then you can take as much as 40-50 percent calories from carbohydrates, 20-30 percent from protein, and 30 percent from fat.

- Incorporate fat, carbohydrates, and protein in every meal.

- If you are taking the right amount of calories for your level of activity, you should not see any significant decrease in weight.

- Adults need 2,000-3,000 calories a day. Smaller and less active people including women need fewer calories while men required more.

Carbohydrates

- For a 2,000-a-day calories requirement, adult men must consume 240-300 grams of carbs a day while adult women should consume about 100-150 grams of carbohydrates a day and majority of these should be in the form of less processed, less refined foods that are low in glycemic.

- Eat whole grains like brown rice and bulgur wheat in which grains are more intact and in few but more substantial pieces. These are much preferred over wheat flour products with almost the same glycemic index as white flour products.

- Reduce eating foods made with wheat flour and sugar like bread as well as packaged foods like pretzels and chips. Thoroughly avoid products made of high fructose syrup.

- Eat more of sweet potatoes, beans, and winter squashes. As for pasta, cook them al dente and eat them moderately.

Fat

- Out of the 2000 calorie requirement in a day, 600 of these must come from fat (about 57 grams) and in a ratio of 1:2:1 of saturated to monounsaturated to polyunsaturated fat.

- You can reduce your consumption of saturated fat by eating less high-fat cheese, butter, unskinned chicken, products made of palm kernel oil, and fatty meats. Also, avoid oils extracted from sunflower, cottonseed, corn and mixed vegetables and take margarine out of your meals.

- Avoid all products with propert

- ies of hydrogenates oils of any kind. Instead, include in your diet nuts and avocados, mainly cashew, almonds, walnuts, and nut butter made from such nuts.

- For your primary cooking oil, use extra-virgin olive oil or coconut butter and if you want neutral-tasting crude, choose expeller-pressed organic canola oil. Pressed versions of natural, high oleic expeller of sunflower and safflower oil can be your second option.

- For your omega-3 fatty acids, choose fresh, frozen wild or canned sockeye salmon, black cod (butterfish and sablefish), sardines packed in olive oil or water. Omega-3 fortified eggs; hemp seed, flax seeds or you may also take fish oil supplement. For this, look for products that provide both DHA and EPA in a convenient daily dosage of 2-3 grams).

Protein

- Your daily intake of protein must be between 80-120 grams but if you have liver or kidney problem, autoimmune disease or allergies, take less protein.

- Consume more of proteins from vegetables, especially from soybeans to be more particular while lessening your consumption of animal protein with the exclusion of fish and high-quality natural cheese and yogurt.

Fiber

- Consume 40 grams of fiber in a day by increasing your consumption of fruits like berries, whole grains, and vegetables especially beans.

- Ready-made cereals are also enriched with good fiber but make sure that it gives you at least 4-5 grams of bran per ounce of serving by reading the label.

Phytonutrients

- To maximize protection against age-related illnesses including cardiovascular disease, neurodegenerative disease, and cancer plus toxins from the environment, consume as many fruits, vegetables, and mushrooms as you can.

- Choose organic produce whenever possible. Learn which conventionally grown crops are most likely to carry pesticide residues and avoid them.

- Regularly eat cruciferous vegetables daily. Examples are vegetables from the cabbage family. Also, include soy in your diet.

- Prefer to drink tea instead of coffee especially the excellent quality white or green oolong tea.

- Consume dark chocolate in moderate amount and with a minimum cocoa content of 70 percent.)

- When drinking alcohol, choose the red wine.

Vitamins and Minerals

Eating a diet consisting of fresh foods or cooked from fresh vegetables is the best way to obtain all your daily requirements of vitamins, minerals, and micronutrients needed by your body. For maximum health and protection, supplement your diet with the following antioxidants.

- 200 milligrams of Vitamin C daily

- For Vitamin E, have 400 IU of natural mixed tocopherols (d-alpha-tocopherol with other tocopherols, or a minimum of 80 milligrams of natural mixed tocopherols and tocotrienols for better result).

- 10,000-15,000 IU of mixed carotenoid daily

- Selenium, 200 micrograms of yeast-bound organic form

- Women must take 500-700 milligram of supplemental calcium like calcium citrate daily depending on their dietary intake of this mineral while men must avoid additional calcium.

- Antioxidants can be likewise most conveniently taken as part of a daily multivitamin or multimineral supplement that also provides 400 micrograms of folic acid and 2,000 IU of vitamin D. It must not contain any amount of iron unless you're a female with regular menstrual periods and no preformed Vitamin A (retinol). Consume these supplements along with your most substantial meal.

Other Dietary Supplements

- If you are not fond of eating oily fish which you must have at least twice a week, take supplemental fish oil either in liquid or capsule form, about 2-3 grams daily of a product containing both DHA and EPA. Find products that are molecularly distilled and certified to be free of heavy metals and other contaminants.

- If you aren't regularly eating turmeric or ginger, consider taking them in supplemental form and when you are prone to metal oil syndrome, take alpha-lipoic acid, about 100-400 milligrams daily.

- Add coenzyme Q10 (CoC10) to your daily regimen: 60-100 milligrams of soft gel form taken with your most substantial meal.

Water

- Drink water liberally or drinks with high water content like tea, lemon water, or a much-diluted fruit juice throughout the day.

- Either use bottled water or have a water purifier in your home to protect yourself from contaminants.

Common Mistakes

It's quite heartbreaking to see people trying to heal themselves from pain and inflammation. They try their best to test every possible diet that promises treatment, but unintentionally take a couple of wrong turns which all end up sabotaging their initial efforts. For people who want to get back to the right lane, here are some of those frequent mistakes people usually commit when trying to follow an anti-inflammatory diet.

Mistake #1 − Not Giving Attention to Food Sensitivity

Most people have some chronic, inflammatory condition (thyroid disorders, autoimmune disease, adrenal dysfunction, digestive issues, skin conditions, and cognitive or mood issues). Food sensitivities need to be identified and addressed to help in their healing process.

While many are trying to get into the diet for treatment of inflammation, still about 90 percent can't get away with gluten or cow's milk sometimes both. These make excuses in the form of calling themselves "Gluten light" or "I don't eat much dairy." But a little amount of food that you are sensitive to will undoubtedly spark off inflammation.

Saying it bluntly, if you keep on eating a little bit of this and that, you will never see any improvement at all regardless of your diet. Foods that are likely to throw off your treatment must be eliminated for a minimum of two weeks though ideally for 4-6 weeks for you to be able to determine if you are reacting.

Mistake #2 – Focusing Only on Food Sensitivity

On the other hand, some people are overly focused on eliminating foods they are sensitive to but not rebalancing their diet. Especially true to gluten and though gluten is a big deal for many, entirely keeping gluten from your diet, it is not altogether the solution to wellness.

When you intend to get away from gluten, you tend to search the gluten-free aisle of a grocery store for every processed gluten-free cookie, frozen gluten-free pizza or any other processed gluten-free food you can find.

When you are desperate to calm acute inflammation, and you know that eliminating certain foods can do that. You are replacing them with other foods that are not ideal either – though packaged and processed foods can be used for a short time. Especially for people whose lifestyle isn't conducive to preparing and cooking whole meals and if the diet requires a drastic shift from their eating lifestyle.

Therefore while trying to find quick fixes, to see positive results especially in the long run, you need to switch your focus to balancing the rest of your diet.

Mistake #3 – Being Afraid of Fat & Calories

A lot of people managed their health by strictly controlling the number of fats and calorie consumption. Though some have genuine concern over fat intake concerning heart disease despite reports dispelling the myth about dietary fat – including saturated fat – being related to increased cardiovascular risk others holds on to their belief that letting go of calories is synonymous with having a healthy weight. When you have some chronic conditions like digestive issues, and you go on an extremely low-calorie diet, this can aggravate your medical situation. Therefore, you need to get out of this kind of mindset. Take note that nutrient-dense foods feed the significant volume of cells that our bodies contain. They likewise act as GPS guiding you a healthy weight and better overall wellness. These foods are apt to fill your appetite and change your taste for the better such as lessening cravings for refined carbs, sugar, and processed foods.

Fat helps in regulating your blood sugar, promotes tissue healing, increase satiety, and boosts immune function. Even your brain is made up of 60 percent fat. With all these, good health is not as absolute as calories in and out. Lifestyle practices and different nutrients direct different hormones and other physiological processes in our bodies. These determine how our body works, how we burn carbohydrates, and how we store fats.

So the good news is this! It means, putting an end to steamed veggies or eating dry chicken breast. You can enjoy eating organic chicken thigh and egg yolk, too! Another thing, veggies are indeed delicious and satisfying when prepared with edible fats and oils. Fat-soluble vitamins A, D, E, and K contained in vegetables, and other nutrient-dense foods are only absorbed by the body when you eat it along with fat.

Therefore, seeking out the good stuff is as crucial as avoiding the bad ones!

Mistake #4 – Not Taking Supplements Consistently

Getting nutrients from what we eat is ideal, but even if how much you count on your daily dietary requirement, issues with soil producing agricultural products having fewer nutrients compared to what it should contain initially are depriving our body needs. Added to these are underlying conditions that make it hard for your body to absorb nutrients like digestive issues and genetic variations. So, there are times when supplements become a vital component of healing any chronic condition.

Supplements can help alleviate digestive symptoms including the treatment of a leaky gut, lowering inflammation, detoxifying, balancing hormones, and replenishing nutrient deficiencies and imbalance. All these are roots of illnesses.

While lots of people are on the supplement, it's sad to know that majority are not good at taking them regularly. Meaning, most of them would make almost all kinds of supplements they have at home for once and forget all about them the next day or the rest of the week. It takes several days before they can remember that they should make another set of these multivitamins or whatever vitamins or mineral supplement they need.

Reactions or effects of these supplements are cumulative and not immediate, and they won't work unless taken on a regular basis. Supplements need time and consistency to work out efficiently.

The need of one individual may differ from that of the others based on specific conditions and current nutritional level that a professional healthcare provider is strongly recommended especially for those with severe medical conditions. However, a useful starting point for those with chronic inflammatory diseases is consuming whole foods, multi-vitamin or multi-mineral, a multi-strain probiotic, or high-vitamin cod level oil. Check with your physician if you are taking blood-thinning medication and try algal oil instead of a vegan substitute.

Mistake #5 – Constantly Changing Diet

Diets have become popular over the decade that many had treated them as a fad rather than a lifestyle or treatment process. Most are into self-diagnosis and readily change their diet and or supplement regime every time they are introduced into a new one.

It's easy to read resources or hear stories from someone and relate yourself to what they are experiencing and then start changing your current diet just because you feel you are in the same situation. But definitely, there's nothing as one strategy that fits all, and when you continuously change the variables, you're making it more difficult to ascertain what works for you. If you feel right about a diet plan, then stick to it and give it enough time to work its magic!

Let's remember that our body is complicated and that sometimes one system needs to be fully healed before it moves on to other parts. When you think you are not making any changes, it is because you are not consistent with your original plan.

Mistake #6 – Not Acknowledging Chronic Stress Role in Healing

Diet does have a significant role in your treatment, but if you don't manage stress efficiently, reparation is almost impossible!

Once you have chronic stress, cortisol or stress hormones are continually rippling through your body and suppressing your immune system resulting in digestive issues such as gut permeability, increase in weight, and causes systemic inflammation. And because we are constantly bombarded with various stressors relating to our daily life, we can't get away from them. Hence, it is vital that we need to find ways to manage stress.

Mistake #7 – Not Having the Right Action Plan

The lack of an action plan or not having the right one can get you off the track in some ways.

"I'm going to eat less after the holidays!"

An example of a vague goal as you are not specific with the kind of result you want to obtain out of it. It would be hard to map out a plan based on this type of goal. If you 're going to achieve something, be specific and definite with your expectations and to reach whatever purpose you have without getting overwhelmed, have a plan and break it down into clear and achievable steps that will somehow motivate you to keep going.

Making your plan too ambitious and unsustainable won't work primarily in the long run. Take, for instance, doing a two-week cleanse that ends up in a feast. When you set up goals that aren't in line with your willingness or readiness to make a shift, then you're destined to burn or crash before seeing its final effect. Your brain releases dopamine, the happy and motivational hormone every time you achieve your goal, regardless of whether it is small or large. Conversely, when you fail, there is a reduction in dopamine which kills your motivation.

Thus, it makes sense to make a plan that is not impossible to achieve and feasible enough to be broken into small actionable steps that will lead you to a satisfactory result.

CHAPTER 4 – THE ULTIMATE DIET PLAN AGAINST INFLAMMATION

Many diseases involve inflammation since it's our body's natural response when it comes to injury or damage. Arthritis, sprained ankle, sinuses, and asthma are but few of them. It is vital for you to know that certain foods will alleviate inflammation. Whether you eat them when you experience soreness or merely put them on your daily diet, one thing's for sure—they help your body in a lot of ways.

Diets filled with fruits and vegetables are packed with anti-oxidants that can significantly help you limit inflammation. Listed below are 21 antioxidant-packed recipes for breakfast, lunch, and dinner for seven days.

Just pick among these 21 recipes your meals for the day and your set to face a pain-free life ahead!

Breakfast

Recipe #1 – Blueberry & Ricotta Oatmeal

As we all know, blueberries are rich in antioxidants. This quick and easy recipe dish benefits both your health and your palate.

Ingredients

- ½ cup of blueberries

- ¼ cup of ricotta cheese, low-fat

- ¾ cup of steel-cut oatmeal, cooked

- 1 ½ tbsp. of almonds, slivered

- 18g (or 2 scoops) of protein powder

Procedure

1. Get your oatmeal and mix in the protein powder.

2. Put the mixture into the serving bowl and add the blueberries.

3. Microwave it for about 2 minutes.

4. Add the ricotta as well as the slivered almonds.

Recipe #2 – Hash & Tomatoes Morning Treat

Easy to prepare and chew, this breakfast recipe bursts with nutrients and flavors.

Ingredients

- 3 oz. of cooked beef sirloin steak (or any meat), minced

- 2 tomatoes, sliced

- 1 Orange

- 2 tbsps. of green pepper, minced

- 3 tbsps. of onion, minced

- 3 tbsps. of mushrooms, minced

- ¼ cup of cooked steel-cut oats

- ½ tsp. of extra virgin olive oil

- 1 tsp. of Worcestershire sauce

- Salt

- Pepper

Procedure

1. Prepare your pan by applying cooking spray on it and place it over a medium flame.

2. Sauté the onions, mushrooms and green peppers in olive oil until they're tender.

3. Add the minced meat as well as the cooked steel-cut oats.

4. Mix in the spices and the Worcestershire sauce.

5. Stir and let it cook for several minutes.

6. Transfer to a plate then add the tomatoes and orange.

Recipe #3 – Crab and Cheese Omelet Breakfast Delight

The combination of crab meat, cheese, oats, and fruits for this meal ensures an excellent morning for you. The anti-inflammatory properties of the fruits and oats vouch for beauty and health in one diet meal.

Ingredients

- 1 oz. of crab meat, canned

- ½ slice of low-fat Pepper Jack Cheese

- 2/3 cup of steel cut oats, cooked

- ½ cup of egg beaters, whites

- ¼ cup of blueberries

- 1/3 banana, chunked

- ½ tsp. of cinnamon

- 2 tbsps. of Peanut Butter

- Stevia

Procedure

1. Put the crabmeat and egg beaters into a bowl and mix.

2. Prepare skillet by spraying olive oil and putting it over medium-high flame.

3. Pour the egg mixture into the skillet and top it with cheese slices.

4. Meanwhile, warm the blueberries, banana chunks, cinnamon, and oats in the microwave.

5. Mix in the peanut butter and stevia.

6. Take note that the heat from the oatmeal melts the banana chunks. Serve and enjoy.

Recipe #4 – Simple Avocado Toast with Egg

Eggs can be an excellent source of different nutrients including protein, B12, omega-3 fats and selenium. Selenium is an antioxidant that protects the cells from being damaged due to inflammation. On top of that, this healthy meal accompanied by spinach and avocados which are also rich sources of antioxidants.

Ingredients

- 1 egg, poached or scrambled

- ½ of an avocado, sliced

- A handful of spinach

- 1-2 slice/s of toasted bread (preferably gluten-free)*

- 1½ tsp. of ghee

- Red pepper flakes

(*_Note_: Feel free to add an extra slice if you prefer it sandwich style.)

Procedure

1. Top the toasted bread with ghee.

2. Add the avocado slices on the toast and top them with spinach.

3. Add the poached or scrambled egg on top of the spinach leaves and sprinkle it with red pepper flakes. Serve and enjoy!

Recipe #5 – Avocado-Raspberry Smoothie

Now, you may find the combination of avocado and raspberry quite peculiar, but the creaminess of avocado makes up for the sour taste of the raspberry. Both provide high quantities of antioxidants, fiber and vitamin C to strengthen immunity and promote wellness.

Ingredients

- 1 avocado, pitted and peeled

- ½ cup of raspberries

- ¾ cup of orange juice

- ¾ cup of raspberry juice

Procedure

1. Just mix all the ingredients in the blender and process.

2. Transfer to a tall glass and serve.

Recipe #6 – Oat – Wheat Tabbouleh

Ingredients

- 1/4 cup old-fashioned rolled oats

- 1/8 cup bulgur wheat

- 1/4 kiwi, peeled and diced

- 2 tablespoon chopped fresh Italian parsley

- 1 tablespoon chopped pecans or almonds

- 1/8 cup diced strawberries

- 1/2 teaspoon chopped fresh mint

- salt and freshly ground pepper to taste

Procedure

1. Combine steel cut oats and bulgur wheat with salt to taste in a large bowl and pour in boiling water, enough to cover them. Let sit for about 45 minutes then pass through a strainer to drain. Press the oats and wheat against the strainer using the back of the

spoon to extract water before transferring to the bowl.

2. Combine all the remaining ingredients and whisk together. Add the oats and wheat and toss. Let sit another 10-15 minutes in the fridge before serving.

Recipe #7 – Blueberry Oatmeal

Ingredients

- 1 cup gluten-free quick-cooking oats

- 1 cup skim milk

- 1/4 cup raw honey

- 1/2 tsp. pure vanilla extract

- 1/2 tsp. ground cinnamon

- 1 tbsp. sliced almonds

- 3/4 cup fresh or frozen blueberries

Procedure

1. Place a saucepan over medium heat. Add the milk and bring to boil

2. Add the oats and cook for about 2 minutes while stirring occasionally.

3. Add honey, vanilla, and cinnamon then blends well.

4. Serve oatmeal in bowls topped with blueberries.

Lunch

Recipe #1 – Mediterranean Tuna Salad

This lunch recipe gives a burst of freshness and isn't too heavy for the stomach. Packed with the healthy goodness of herbs and spices, it's one cool lunch treat for you. Feel free to serve it with toast, crackers or pita bread.

Ingredients

- 2 x 5oz. can tuna flakes in water, drained

- 2 large tomatoes*

- ¼ cup of kalamata or mixed olives, chopped

- 2 tbsp. of red peppers, roasted on fire and cut

- 2 tbsp. of fresh basil, chopped

- 2 tbsp. of red onion, minced

- ¼ cup of mayonnaise

- 1 tbsp. fresh lemon juice

- 1 tbsp. capers

- Salt

- Pepper

*_Note_: Instead of tomatoes, you can also choose bread slices to make a tuna sandwich. Pita bread, greens, toasts and crackers can also be your choice of alternatives.

Procedure

1. Mix all the ingredients (except the tomatoes) into a large salad bowl. See to it that they're well combined.

2. Slice the tomatoes into sixths, creating a flower-like design. Be careful not to cut all the way through the bottom.

3. Gently open the slices and scoop the tuna salad right into the center of the tomato.

Recipe #2 – Quinoa Salad Tropical Treat

Ingredients

- 1 cup of dried quinoa, rinsed

- 3 cups of Romaine lettuce*, roughly chopped

- required avocado, chopped or thinly sliced

- 1 large mango, skinned, pitted and chopped

- 1 cup of apple or carrot, finely chopped

- 1 cup cashews, coarsely chopped

- ½ red onion, finely chopped

- ¼ cup of mint, finely chopped

- ½-inch of ginger, finely chopped

- 2 tbsp. of honey or agave

- 1 tbsp. of extra-virgin olive oil

- juice of 1 lime

- freshly ground black pepper

- 1 tbsp. of sea salt

*_Note_: You can also use your own choice of greens.

Procedure

1. For the quinoa, boil 2 cups of water in a medium saucepan. Add the quinoa and let it simmer. Cover the pan for about 15-20 minutes and remove from heat. Let the quinoa cool.

2. Meanwhile, toss the chopped apple (or carrot) and red onions in a large bowl.

3. In a different bowl, whisk the olive oil, lime juice, and honey together. Add the mixture along with the apple and onions.

4. Add the cooled quinoa and the chopped mango to the bowl and toss.

5. Add the cilantro, ginger, and mint. Season with salt and pepper.

6. Scoop the mixture over the Romaine lettuce (or choice of greens). Chill before serving, or you can serve it at room temperature.

Recipe #3 – Marinated Beet & Apple Salad

Beets and apples are considered a powerhouse when it comes to foods rich in antioxidants. They can help you repair muscle fibers and boost your immune system. This particular recipe isn't only a health-friendly meal but is also palate-friendly.

Ingredients

- 4 medium beets, washed

- 1 Granny Smith Apple, chopped

- 1 large banana pepper, chopped

- ¼ cup of red wine vinegar

- 1 tsp. of Worcestershire sauce*

- ¼ cup of olive or avocado oil

- ¼ tsp. of dry mustard

- ¼ cup of coconut sugar or raw sugar

- ¼ cup of pecan or walnuts, chopped

- ¼ tsp. of sea salt

- ¼ tsp. of black pepper

- ¼ tsp. of onion salt (optional)

*_Note_: If you're a vegan, you can substitute Tamari Sauce + ¼ tsp. apple cider vinegar for the Worcestershire sauce.

Procedure

1. Put 1 inch of water and a dash of sea salt in a large pot and put over medium-high flame. Place the beets in the steamer basket and steam for about 20 minutes.

2. Once the beets have softened, peel them and chop into quarters.

3. In a large mixing bowl, mix the apple, banana peppers, and the beets then set aside.

4. In a small mixing bowl, incorporate the sugar, salt, and other seasonings then set aside.

5. Drizzle the beets-apple-pepper mixture with vinegar, oil and Worcestershire sauce (or Tamari).

6. Add the seasoning mixture and toss well.

7. Refrigerate the salad for about 8-24 hours to marinate.

8. Before serving, add walnuts or pecans and any seasoning you want.

Recipe #4 – Pan-seared Salmon on Baby Arugula Salad

If you're looking for a sharp flavor, baby arugula can humor your palate.

Ingredients

For the salmon:

- 2 x 6 oz. center-cut salmon fillets

- 1 ½ tbsp. of olive oil

- 1 ½ tbsp. of fresh lemon juice

- Salt

- Freshly ground black pepper

For the salad:

- 3 cups of baby arugula leaves

- 2/3 cup of grape or cherry tomatoes, halved

- ¼ cup of red onion, thinly slivered

- 1 tbsp. of red-wine vinegar

- 1 tbsp. of extra-virgin olive oil

- Salt

- Freshly ground black pepper

Procedure

1. Put the salmon fillets in a shallow bowl. Add the salt, pepper, lemon juice and olive oil. Set it aside for about 15 minutes for the flavors to sink in.

2. Place a non-stick skillet over medium-high flame and cook the salmon with the skin side down for about 2-3 minutes.

3. Reduce the heat to medium and cover the pan. Let the salmon for about 3-4 minutes more. Remember that its skin should be crispy and the flesh medium-rare.

4. For the meantime, toss the tomatoes, onion, and arugula in a large salad bowl.

5. Before serving, add the oil, vinegar, salt, and pepper. Toss well and serve.

Recipe #5 – Pumpkin, Chili, and Coconut Soup

A pumpkin is known to be enriched with beta-cryptoxanthin which is a potent anti-inflammatory. Such food is best absorbed by your body when coupled with fat; thus, the oil and cream are crucial ingredients not only to the taste but also for its effectiveness.

Ingredients

For the pumpkin soup:

- 1.2 kg (or 2.6 lbs) of pumpkin, peeled, pitted and cut into 2-inch chunks

- 1 x 165ml can of coconut cream

- 1 long red chili, pitted

- 1 carrot, peeled and cut into 2-inch pieces

- 4 cups of vegetable stock (or chicken stock)

- 1 tsp. of powdered ginger

- 1 tbsp. of vegetable oil

For the garlic croutons:

- 2 slices of day-old white sourdough

- 1 tbsp. of butter

- 1 clove of garlic, halved

Procedure

For the pumpkin soup:

1. Put a large stockpot over medium heat and put 1 tbsp of oil. Cook the carrot and pumpkin chunks for about 3 minutes or until they achieve light brown coloring. Remember to stir while cooking continuously.

2. Add the stock, chili, and ginger. Let it simmer for about 20 minutes or until the carrot, and pumpkin chunks are tender.

3. Take the soup off the heat and blend the soup. If you have a stick blender, it should be perfect for this step.

4. Add the coconut cream, put back the soup into the heat and bring it to a boil.

5. Once it boils, turn off the heat and let it cool for a bit.

For the garlic croutons:

1. Rub the garlic clove on both sides of the bread slices.

2. Chop the bread into 2-centimeter cubes.

3. In a small frying pan, heat the butter until it's bubbly.

4. Add the bread cubes and cook. Continue to stir until the cubes are crispy and light brown.

To serve:

1. Divide the soup into serving bowls with the croutons on the side. Feel free to add an extra drizzle of coconut cream over the top of the soup.

2. Put a handful of croutons into the soup. Bon appetit!

Recipe #6 – Fettuccine with Kale Pesto

Packed with phytonutrients as well as micronutrients, this is certifiably one nutritious meal.

Ingredients

For the pesto:

- 4 cups of kale, stemmed and chopped

- ½ cup of Parmigiano-Reggiano cheese, grated

- ¼ cup of pine nuts

- 6 tbsp. of extra virgin olive oil

- ¼ tsp. of red pepper flakes

- 2 cloves of garlic, chopped

- 1 tsp. of salt

For the pasta:

- 1lb. of fettuccine pasta (or 1 lb. of pappardelle pasta)

- 1 cup (+ more) of Parmigiano-Reggiano cheese, grated

Procedure

For the pesto:

1. Boil a large pot of water. Meanwhile, fill a large bowl with cold water and ice.

2. Plunge the kale into the boiling water and cook for about 3 minutes.

3. Transfer the kale to the ice water using tongs. This process will allow the kale to retain its bright green coloring.

4. After 3 minutes, drain the kale using a colander. Firmly squeeze it to eliminate excess water.

5. Toss the kale and the remaining pesto ingredients into the blender. Process it until you achieve a smooth puree consistency.

6. Transfer the pesto to a container and refrigerate.

For the pasta:

- Boil a large pot of water. Remember to add a bit of salt.

- Add the fettuccine and cook until al dente.

- Before the pasta is done, remove 2 tbsp. of water from the pot and add it to the pesto. Add some cheese and stir well.

- Using the colander, drain the pasta and toss it with pesto. Add more cheese if you want and serve.

Recipe #7 – Fresh and Crunch Broccoli

Perfect recipe for your inflammatory diet! What's more? This versatile recipe can be converted into a sandwich or tortilla to suit your on-the-go schedule.

Ingredients

- 2 cups of broccoli florets

- 2 cups kale, white parts removed and chopped

- 1 of cucumber (about 1 ¾ cups), peeled, seeded and diced

- 2 cups seedless red grapes, cut into quarters

- 1 cup cooked quinoa, cooled*

- ½ cup of small red onion, finely diced

- ½ cup of almonds, slivered

- 2 tbsp. of vegan mayonnaise

- 2 tsp. of apple cider vinegar

- 1 tbsp. of agave nectar

- 1 tsp. of poppy seeds

- 1 ½ tbsp. of lemon juice

- ½ tsp. of ground sea salt

- ¼ tsp. of freshly ground black pepper

*Note: 1/3 cup of dry quinoa can make a cup of cooked quinoa.

Procedure

1. In a large bowl, put the kale, broccoli, cucumber, grapes, quinoa, red onion and almond slivers.

2. In a small bowl, whisk together the mayonnaise, poppy seeds, agave nectar, cider vinegar, lemon juice, salt and ground pepper.

3. Add the salad dressing to the vegetables.

4. Toss until the veggies, and the dressing is well combined. Serve.

Dinner

Recipe #1 – Roasted Salmon with Zucchini, Lemon, and Dill

With zucchini, lemon and dill present, this meal is packed with anti-inflammatory properties that can benefit your health.

Ingredients

- 4 x 8 oz. of salmon fillets, skinless

- 2 lemons, quartered and pitted

- 3 medium zucchini (about 1 ½ lb.), diagonally cut into 1-inch thick slices

- 8 sprigs of fresh dill

- 2 tbsp. of olive oil

- Salt

- Ground pepper

Procedure

1. Heat your broiler, placing it 4 inches above the heat.

2. Incorporate the lemons, dill, and zucchini in a large-rimmed, broiler-proof baking sheet.

3. Drizzle the mixture with oil; and season with salt and ground pepper. Toss well to coat everything.

4. Place the salmon fillets on the veggies and season each with salt and pepper.

5. Broil for about 15-20 minutes or until the veggies are tender and the fish is opaque.

Recipe #2 – Classic Caesar Salad

This recipe packs with top foods for anti-inflammatory diet: oregano, olives, tomatoes, and cucumbers. If you want the Mediterranean style for dinner, then try this one!

Ingredients

- 5 Persian cucumbers

- 12 to 14 small vine-ripened tomatoes, quartered

- 1 small red onion, halved and thinly sliced

- 1 x 4 oz. block Greek feta cheese, packed in brine

- 1 cup kalamata olives, halved and pitted

- ¼ cup of red wine vinegar

- Juice of one lemon + grated zest

- 1 tsp. of dried oregano

- ¼ cup of extra-virgin olive oil (+ more for drizzling)

- 1 tsp. of honey

- Kosher salt

- Freshly ground pepper

- Fresh oregano leaves, for topping (optional)

Procedure

1. In a bowl of heavily salted ice water, soak the red onions for about 15 minutes.

2. In a large bowl, combine the vinegar, dried oregano, honey, half a teaspoon of salt, a quarter teaspoon of pepper, lemon juice, and zest.

3. Gently stir in the olive oil slowly until it's thoroughly combined with the mixture.

4. Add the olives and tomatoes then toss.

5. Meanwhile, peel the cucumbers, creating an alternating green strip design. Don't forget to cut the ends, cut them into halves lengthwise and slice crosswise for about half an inch thickness.

6. Add the cucumbers to the bowl.

7. Drain the red onions, add to the bowl and toss to incorporate everything.

8. Drain the feta and cut it horizontally into 4 even rectangles.

9. Transfer the salad to serving plates.

10. Before serving, top them with oregano, feta and a drizzle of olive oil. You can also season with ground pepper.

Recipe #3 – Mediterranean Grilled Lamb Chops with Mint

The anti-inflammatory benefits of mint allow you to prevent indigestion, colitis, flatulence, and IBS (irritable bowel syndrome). Paired with lamb chops, expect a healthy and pleasant dinner with your loved ones.

Ingredients

- 12 small rib (about 2 1/3 lbs.) of lamb chops

- ½ cup (+ more for sprinkling) of fresh mint leaves, chopped

- ⅓ cup of extra-virgin olive oil

- ¼ tsp. of red pepper flakes

- 2 cloves garlic, smashed

- Sea salt

Procedure

1. Preheat your grill into medium-high.

2. In a medium bowl, combine: chopped mint leaves, red pepper flakes, salt and olive oil.

3. Rub the lamb chops with garlic. Remember to rub them all over.

4. Transfer a few tablespoons of mint mixture into a small bowl and use this to brush on the lamb chops.

5. Grill the lamb chops for about 3-4 minutes per side. Go medium-rare. To test, press the middle part of the lamb chop with your finger. If it's slightly firm, then it's medium-rare.

6. Transfer the chops to the platter and brush them some more with the mint mixture.

7. Sprinkle them with mint and serve with the remaining mint mixture on the side.

Recipe #4 – Broccoli Rabe with Cherry Peppers

Broccoli rabe or rapini, just like its cousin, broccoli, is a superfood. It is packed with vitamins A, B, C, K, iron, potassium, calcium, magnesium, zinc and omega-3 fatty. It has cancer-fighting and anti-inflammatory properties that can aid your body to stay healthy and healthy.

Ingredients

- 2 bunches of broccoli rabe

- ¼ cup of cherry peppers or pimiento in a jar, sliced

- 2 tbsp. of liquid from cherry pepper jar

- 1 tbsp. of olive oil

- 2 cloves of garlic, sliced

- Parmesan cheese shaved

- Salt

- Pepper

Procedure

1. Steam the broccoli rabe for about 7 minutes or until tender.

2. While steaming, put a saucepan over medium flame and heat the olive oil.

3. Add the garlic cloves and cook until golden.

4. Mix in the cherry peppers and 2 tbsp. of liquid from its container.

5. Toss in the broccoli rabe then seasons with salt and pepper.

6. Finally, drizzle it with olive oil and sprinkle with shaved parmesan cheese.

Recipe #5 – Baked Tilapia with Pecan Rosemary Topping

Tilapia is an excellent source of selenium, a mineral with antioxidant properties which can help protect cells from damage. Pair this dish with gluten-free bread, and you're in for a healthier dinner!

Ingredients

- 4 x 4 oz. tilapia fillets

- ⅓ cup of raw pecans, chopped

- 2 tsp. of fresh rosemary, chopped

- ⅓ cup of panko breadcrumbs

- 1 egg white

- ½ tsp. of brown sugar

- 1 pinch of cayenne pepper

- 1½ tsp olive oil

- ⅛ tsp. of salt

Instructions

1. Preheat your oven to 350°F.

2. Stir the breadcrumbs, pecans, cayenne pepper, sugar and salt together in a small baking dish.

3. Add olive oil and toss to coat everything.

4. Bake the pecan mixture for about 7-8 minutes or until it's golden brown.

5. Next, increase heat to 400°F and apply cooking spray to a large glass baking dish.

6. In a different shallow dish, whisk the egg white.

7. Dip the tilapia fillets by dipping them one piece at a time in the egg white and then the pecan mixture. Coat each side evenly.

8. Place the fillets in the glass baking dish.

9. Place and press the remaining pecan mixture on the top of the fillets.

10. Bake for about 10 minutes and serve hot.

Recipe #6 – Grilled Tuna Steaks With Strawberry-Mango Salsa

Strawberries earned its spot as one of the foods rich in antioxidants while mangoes are right for your digestion. Both are packed with vitamins and minerals our body needs. Meanwhile, tuna is an excellent source of antioxidant Omega-3 fatty acids. Bring them all together in one sumptuous meal, and you have one fabulous dinner.

Ingredients

For the tuna:

- 1½ lbs. of tuna steaks

- 1 tbsp. of olive oil

For the salsa:

- ⅔ cup of strawberries, diced

- ⅔ cup of mango, diced

- 3 tbsp. of fresh cilantro, chopped

- 2 tbsp. of red onions, diced

- 1 jalapeno, finely chopped

- 1 clove of garlic, crushed

- 2 tsp. of fresh lime juice

- 1 tbsp. of olive oil

Procedure

1. Heat your gas grill to medium heat.

2. While waiting for your grill, brush the tuna steaks with olive oil and set aside.

3. For the salsa, add the strawberries, mangoes, garlic, and onions in a bowl and toss.

4. Add the cilantro, jalapeno, oil and lime juice.

5. Once the grill is already hot, cook the tuna steaks for about 6-8 minutes per side.

6. Remove the tuna steaks from the grill and transfer to serving plates.

7. Before serving, top each steak with strawberry-mango salsa. Enjoy!

Recipe #7 – Curried Veggies with Poached Egg

Despite the heavenly goodness of eggs, the real star player for this recipe is the curried vegetables. The garlic, chickpeas, zucchini, carrots, and cauliflower contain anti-inflammatory properties that protect our overall health and boost our immune system.

Ingredients

- 4 fresh eggs

- 1 x 14 oz. can of chickpeas (or garbanzo beans), drained

- ¼ head of cauliflower, roughly chopped

- 2 carrots, cut into rounds

- 1 zucchini, chopped

- 1 small onion, diced

- 3 cloves of garlic, minced

- 1 cup of plain tomato sauce

- 2 tsp. of curry powder

- ½ tsp. of ginger

- ½ tsp. of cumin

- 1 cup of water

- 2 tbsp. olive oil

- Salt

- Pepper

- Parsley or cilantro, for garnish

Procedure

1. Place saucepan over medium flame and heat the oil. Sauté the onions for about 3 minutes and add the garlic. Continue sautéing both for another 2 minutes.

2. Toss in the cauliflower, chickpeas, and carrots. Continue to sauté for another 4-5 minutes.

3. Mix in the zucchini as well as the spices. Cook for another 3 minutes until you can smell the aroma emitted by the spices.

4. Stir in the tomato sauce and water. Cover the saucepan with lid and allow the mixture to simmer until the cauliflower has become tender.

5. Next, carefully crack each egg into the pan. Be careful so that you won't break the yolk. Remember —do not stir!

6. Cover again with lid and let the eggs be cooked according to your desired level of doneness.

7. Carefully transfer into serving bowls and garnish each with cilantro (or parsley). You can also add your favourite hot sauce if you want to. Enjoy!

CONCLUSION

Our body is a perfect machine with a built-in resistor from harmful external factors as well as self-healing ability, which is inflammation. However, along with modern living, progress, and technology, the food chain was significantly affected and so is our ecology and natural life. Industrial waste had brought harm to our soil, taking away its natural elements that provide nutrients to every plant species that depend on it. Even animals that rely on nature were deprived of their provisional nutrients which in effect likewise affect the food that we eat.

Plants and animals had long provided us with all the natural elements and nutrients that our body needs. Unfortunately, their weak state became our deficit regarding nutrient-enriched sources. Furthermore, because of our need for mass production, fewer people are indulging in the natural production of food. Hence our inflammation process, which is the self-healing function of our body turned chaotic that instead of healing the body, it becomes destructive.

To save our body from more harm and get inflammation back to its normal process, we must learn how to protect our body from more damage and eat the right diet can put everything back to the right places. When the body is strong and healthy, we don't need to be bothered by illnesses and health condition as our body knows what's best for us.

Through this book, we are hoping that we had provided you with adequate knowledge on how inflammation works in our body and how we can prevent negative responses of inflammation. With the right plan and diet like what we have provided you in this book, we believe that you can live a healthier and happier life!

FINAL WORDS

Thank you again for purchasing this book! I really hope this book is able to help you.

The next step is for you to **join our email newsletter** to receive updates on any upcoming new book releases or promotions. You can sign-up for free and as a bonus, you will also receive our "*7 Fitness Mistakes You Don't Know You're Making*" book! This bonus book breaks down many of the most common fitness mistakes and will demystify many of the complexities and science of getting into shape. Having all this fitness knowledge and science organized into an actionable step-by-step book will help you get started in the right direction in your fitness journey! To join our free email newsletter and grab your free book, please visit the link and signup: **www.hmwpublishing.com/gift**

Finally, if you enjoyed this book, then I would like to ask you for a favor, would you be kind enough to leave a review for this book? It would be greatly appreciated!

Thank you and good luck in your journey!

ABOUT THE CO-AUTHOR

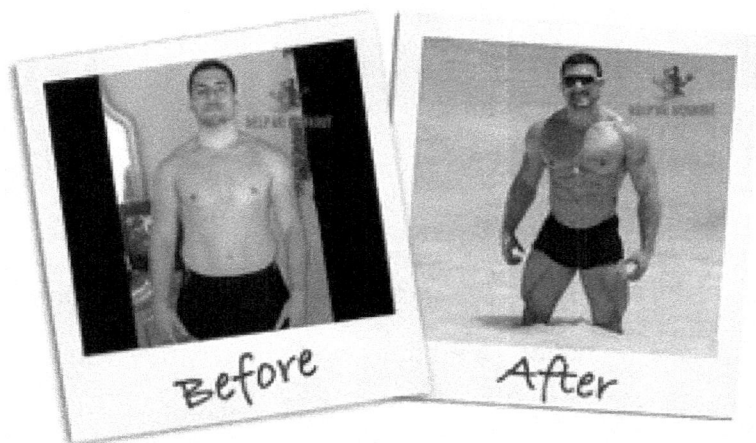

Before After

My name is George Kaplo; I'm a certified personal trainer from Montreal, Canada. I'll start off by saying I'm not the biggest guy you will ever meet and this has never really been my goal. In fact, I started working out to overcome my biggest insecurity when I was younger, which was my self-confidence. This was due to my height measuring only 5 foot 5 inches (168cm), it pushed me down to attempt anything I ever wanted to achieve in life. You may be going through some challenges right now, or you may simply want to get fit, and I can certainly relate.

For me personally, I was always kind of interested in the health & fitness world and wanted to gain some muscle due to the numerous bullying in my teenage years about my height and my overweight body. I figured I couldn't do anything about my height, but I sure can do something about how my body looked like. This was the beginning of my transformation journey. I had no idea where to start, but I just got started. I felt worried and afraid at times that other people would make fun of me for doing the exercises the wrong way. I always wished I had a friend that was next to me who was knowledgeable enough to help me get started and "show me the ropes."

After a lot of work, studying and countless trial and errors. Some people began to notice how I was getting more fit and how I was starting to form a keen interest in the topic. This led many friends and new faces to come to me and ask me for fitness advice. At first, it seemed odd when people asked me to help them get in shape. But what kept me going is when they started to see changes in their own body and told me it's the first time that they saw real results!

From there, more people kept coming to me, and it made me realize after so much reading and studying in this field that it did help me but it also allowed me to help others. I'm now a fully certified personal trainer and have trained numerous clients to date who have achieved amazing results.

Today, my brother Alex Kaplo (also a Certified Personal Trainer) and I own & operate this publishing venture, where we bring passionate and expert authors to write about health and fitness topics. We also run an online fitness website "HelpMeWorkout.com" and I would love to connect with by inviting you to visit the website on the following page and signing up to our e-mail newsletter (you will even get a free book).

Last but not least, if you are in the position I was once in and you want some guidance, don't hesitate and ask... I'll be there to help you out!

Your friend and coach,

George Kaplo
Certified Personal Trainer

Get another book for Free

I want to thank you for purchasing this book and offer you another book (just as long and valuable as this book), "Health & Fitness Mistakes You Don't Know You're Making", completely free.

Visit the link below to signup and receive it:

www.hmwpublishing.com/gift

In this book, I will break down the most common health & fitness mistakes, you are probably committing right now, and I will reveal how you can easily get in the best shape of your life!

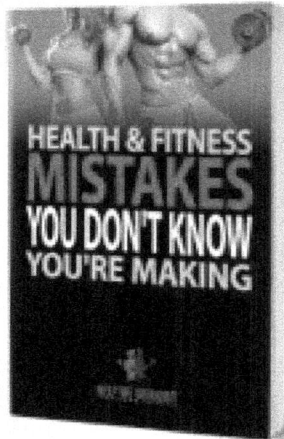

In addition to this valuable gift, you will also have an opportunity to get our new books for free, enter giveaways, and receive other valuable emails from me. Again, visit the link to sign up:

www.hmwpublishing.com/gift

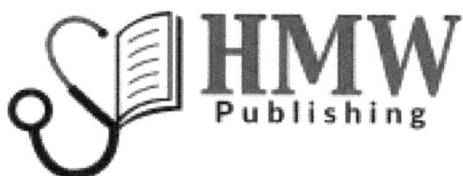

For more great books visit:

HMWPublishing.com

www.ingramcontent.com/pod-product-compliance
Lightning Source LLC
Chambersburg PA
CBHW071114030426
42336CB00013BA/2080